Build Muscle Faster with Blood Flow Restriction Training

How to Build Muscle Faster, Safer and Easier with BFR/Kaatsu/Occlusion Training

Table of Contents

Book Description

Ease of Use of BFR

The Necessity of BFR

Chapter 1: What is BFR and How It Works

Advancement in Musculoskeletal Rehabilitation

The Strategy behind the Muscle Strengthening

Exercising with BFR

Chapter 2: Differences Between BFR and Conventional Training

Key Differences between BFR and Conventional Methods

Conventional Method of Weight Training

The Simplicity of the BFR Method of Strength Training

Chapter 3: Benefits

Specific Advantages of BFR Method

Physiology Involved in BFR

Action of Restriction

Increased Growth of Muscle Cells

Wow! Congratulations!

Chapter 4: Workout Training Protocol and Correct Posture

Determine the Cuff Pressure

List of Exercises to Do

Dumbbell Flat Chest Press

Dumbbell Incline Chest Press

Do Push-ups

Chest Flyes

One Arm Row

Leg Curl

Dumbbell Curls

Overhead Dumbbell Extension

Quarter Squat

Stiff-Legged Deadlift

Chapter 5: Risks and contradictions

Set the Safe BFR Band Pressure

More Contraindications and Rare Side Effects

Use of BFR for the Elderly

Reflection on KAATSU

The Action of BFR on the Cardiovascular System

Dealing with Blood Clots

BFR and the Nervous System

Chapter 6: BFR Equipment

Picking the Right Size Cuff

Chapter 7: Where to Buy Equipment

Conclusion

Thank you!

Bibliography

Introduction

Many of us wish we had a strong body with outstanding muscles and some of us work to achieve it. But, do we use the right method? Here in this book, *"Build Muscle Faster with Blood Flow Restriction Training,"* you will discover the secret method of using light weights and achieving impossible results.

So, what is BFR? In the Blood Flow Restriction Training, we use one quarter or one-third of the weights used on conventional training methods. Does this work? Yes, because we use BFR bands during training to "trick" the body into thinking it is lifting huge weights. "That is a laugh because it is not going to work," you say.

In reality, it works and we witness it in real life. Dr. Yoshiaki Sato is a living testament to the efficacy of BFR training. His huge muscles at the age of 73 show us how dependable it is and his detailed instructions (he is the inventor of the BFR training technique) tell us how to get to the other shore with the least effort. There is hardly any cost involved and assured results await you if you are willing to give it a try.

So, get into the water and start splashing around, it could only make you better. Start on the journey to full fitness with BFR today.

Book Description

BFR ranks among the few undiscovered wonders of the Fitness and Bodybuilding world. Most people prefer to go the long and strenuous route of Conventional Weight Resistance Training and discard Blood Flow Resistance training out of hand. But, it remains one of the most cherished methods of rehabilitation for injured and sick people and the cherry on the pie for the elderly for one reason - it involves small weights!

Ease of Use of BFR

It is not easy for the modern man to spend time away from his work and social life. The use of BFR helps him make light work of the evening or morning gym sessions through the use of bands that amplify his or her workout efforts. The highlights of this are as follows:

- Use of 8 lbs. instead of 30 lbs.
- Increasing reps to improve the impact on the muscles.
- Making use of BFR bands to occlude blood flow.
- More growth hormones for developing muscles with ease.
- A natural process without the use of medication or anything else.

The fact that this method is in use for rehabilitating patients suffering from extreme ailments such as Parkinson's disease and accident injuries is a testimony to its efficacy and its safety.

The Necessity of BFR

One might get tempted to ask, "Why should I do these exercises?" The reason is that fitness is a necessity for us. Some prefer to do full weight exercises while others prefer to ease the pain by opting for the BFR method. Also, this method saves us time which is an important factor.

When you have an interest in developing big (read - huge muscles because that is what happens in this method) and wish to save a lot of trouble, the obvious answer is to check out and use the BFR training method.

Chapter 1: What is BFR and How It Works

The idea of bodybuilding raises visions of heavy weights and sweating bodies involved in lengthy workouts in the gymnasium. Muscle development exercises are, by convention, lengthy and strenuous. But, they did not stay that way for long because of one important development in bodybuilding technology.

Advancement in Musculoskeletal Rehabilitation

Developed by Dr. Yoshiaki Sato, Blood Flow Resistance training, shortened to BFR, is the technique of building muscles without having to indulge in over-energetic mechanisms. Unimaginable but simple, this technique involves the basics of muscle building and offers an alternative to flogging yourself out.

Wonderful patient recovery in rehab.

What is remarkable about BFR is its efficacy with patient rehabilitation. In a controlled study, the volume, cross-sectional area of the thigh muscles and quadriceps, tests for knee extension, leg press, and muscle strength along with Multistage Locomotion Test and Y-Balance Test showed remarkable improvement in the control group that underwent the BFR sessions for patients undergoing rehabilitation.

Method of BFR.

During BFR training, arterial inflow is partially restricted while the venous outflow is fully restricted using BFR equipment. By doing this, the strength and muscle mass increases manifold for even single rep at one-third of the max weight one would normally use. This means you do not have to stress yourself lifting the max weight to get the best gain. Using this ideal muscle-strengthening strategy, muscle builders and athletes can gain an enormous amount of muscles in a short time. But, what is more significant is that patients undergoing physiotherapy can speed up their recovery using this BFR technique. Since the elderly and injured need only lift a fraction of the weight, muscle recovery and strength training become easier.

The Strategy behind the Muscle Strengthening

The restriction in the venous blood flow creates a situation where there is low oxygen. This hypoxic environment triggers physiological reactions leading to many benefits for the individual such as:

- Better production of hormones such as IGF-1 and Growth Hormone that make up the group of fitness hormones.
- Stimulating the fast-twitch muscles to kick in and this enhances the volume of muscles.
- There is a significant increase in vascular endothelial growth factor referred to as VEGF. This enhances the growth of blood vessels (very important for the satellite cells) and improves their lining.

The growth of blood vessels in the satellite region helps develop muscle fiber faster and better. Blood vessels help the cells grow and this significant difference helps the user of the BFR method develop bigger muscles.

Oxygen gets depleted through exercise.

To know how this strategy works, one has to know that we have two kinds of muscle fibers in our body. One is the slow-acting Type I fibers that use oxygen and helps improve endurance. The second is Type II that acts fast and is glycolytic, they do not use any oxygen at all. They get the energy they need by producing pyruvate from glucose which then metabolizes into lactate in the absence of oxygen and mitochondria.

When this reaction sets in to produce lactic acid, one experiences burn. This happens for both conventional weight training and BFR methods without any difference. The restricted blood flow causes an accumulation of metabolites. You are not causing total occlusion; blood flow remains reduced to half of the normal arterial occlusion pressure when you do BFR. This is true for both the limbs - hand and leg, you tie the extremities with elastic bands to reduce blood flow.

Interaction of two muscle types.

During the exercise regime, our Type I muscles get exhausted fast. They use all oxygen there is and this creates an anaerobic state in that muscle region. When we exercise more, the energy must come from somewhere. Type I muscle can go on no longer and so the Type II muscles begin to take up the strain. This is because the Type II muscles do not need any oxygen to function.
You can see how muscle fibers begin to grow. We create the ideal conditions for their growth using the elastic bands (devised by Dr. Sato). For the Type II muscle fibers to grow, we need to have more blood flow and create the conditions for the growth of blood vessels which occurs when the fitness hormones begin their work. The growth of excess blood vessels helps stimulate and generate muscle cells in the satellite zone. This region is outside the normal muscle growth zone.

The action of lactic acid build-up

The metabolic and hormonal benefits start when the lactic acid accumulates locally. We witness a huge increase in the size and strength of your muscles, and you can see it because the muscles swell up. The increase in lactic acid levels causes an increase in osmotic pressure and to maintain homeostasis, water rushes to the area. This makes your muscles swell up.

Exercising with BFR

KAATSU training began in Japan five decades ago and it means extra (ka) pressure (atsu). This method uses more repetition with lesser weights meaning you do 30 reps in the place of the 10-12 reps you would always do. The use of lesser weights means you don't have to strain yourself as you would do in conventional training.

Keep control of the blood flow.

Adjust the bands so that it allows the arterial blood through but not the venous blood. This venous blood flows to the heart and by restricting its flow, you deplete the oxygen present in the region. High-intensity weight training can cause serious tissue damage and you circumvent this by lessening the weight you lift.

The trick is to increase the amount of growth hormone secreted and reduce the myostatin that inhibits muscle growth. This helps the muscle cells get their full volume during exercise.

The arrangement involves pressure cuffs and knee wraps to regulate blood flow. This is to allow the blood to enter the muscle through the arterial blood flow while at the top of the limb, a restriction is in place to stop the venous blood from leaving. The occultation of blood resulted in pain observed young Sato when he was a youth. This pain he experienced was in his calves when he sat down in the traditional Japanese sitting position and it was very like that which one experienced when lifting weights.

Reduce pain in the arms and legs.

Having realized that blood flow restriction could increase or decrease pain, young Sato set out to discover the technique we now know as BFR through a series of experiments using elastic bands to restrict blood flow. The mechanism of muscle growth begins with a swelling of the muscle cells. Since one needn't exert oneself, a mere 30-50% of the full power one would always use is enough, a light warm-up is enough.
The traditional KAATSU device is an inflatable cuff that helps you control the pressure of your blood with a high degree of accuracy. Since this is not available for everyone, one can use cotton elastic bandages instead. It is necessary to take care *not* to compress *both* artery and vein when you apply the bandages.
When you exercise, begin with a max rep of about 30 - 35 when your normal rep is about 10 0r 12. Your second rep needn't be the same, a little less will not affect the efficiency of the exercise program.

Chapter 2: Differences Between BFR and Conventional Training

While medical technology is making steady progress in the fields of analysis and treatment of diseases, the practical world of muscle building has seen little development until BFR arrived on the scene. Turning on the muscle-building process by pumping weights and sweating it out is conventional, dependable, and every bodybuilder's first step up in their sandbox. Conventional training is nothing to sneeze at, it is the relevant and honest way forward in the muscle-building process.

When one lifts weights, they create minute tears in the muscle fiber. The trauma triggers a cascade of regenerative reactions within the body and to keep it within tolerable limits, conventional weight trainers use small increments in the load one lifts to stimulate protein synthesis. Satellite cells bind to the damaged cells in their attempt to fix them. It is in the interest of the conventional athlete to do as much damage, by which we mean muscle tears so that the amount of repair is also extensive resulting in big muscle gain.

Key Differences between BFR and Conventional Methods

With Blood Flow Resistance (BFR) training, things change from several perspectives.

1. When working with conventional weight training methods, you lift weights that lie within 60-80% of the most you can lift. Whereas with BFR, you use 0-30% of your best effort only.
2. You will use elastic bands and do more reps in your first attempt in the BFR method.

One can control those pneumatic bands you tie on the extremities of your arm or leg (whichever part you work on) using hand-held KAATSU units. You condition your body differently to get another response than what you will get from conventional strength training.

Why does BFR work?

In BFR, you make your body 'think differently' and so it responds in an enhanced manner. By altering the blood flow pressure, you make the body believe that the condition gets changed enormously. It responds by changing the hormone and growth levels. This leads to an increase in the amount of satellite cell growth. The satellite region is the area adjoining that of your muscles.

In this region, an excess of blood vessels begins to grow as a response to the heightened pressure of the blood flow. Since the constriction you place also leads to a low oxygen environment, as soon as the Type I muscles begin to tire away, Type II muscles take up the load. They don't need oxygen and so they begin to grow.

This doesn't happen in the conventional methods because the entire exercise takes place when there is enough oxygen so Type I muscles will take up the load from your exercise. When the Type II muscles grow, there is an immediate, massive increase in the girth of the muscles in the working region. Because the body thinks that it is lifting a huge weight (the excess pressure makes this ruse work!) it supplies the benefits to counter the adverse situation it faces. We see the first reaction in the way there is a profusion of blood vessels spreading around the region. With plenty of blood, there is extensive growth of tissues.

Conventional Method of Weight Training

Conventional weight training focuses on isolating a group of muscles to enhance its development. For the bodybuilder, the full development of muscles is important. It involves the muscles of the back, chest, arms, legs, abs, and glutes in equal proportion. The athlete or game player is more likely to focus on functional training - the exercise regimen that helps him or her develop speed, agility, or power in the arms, and things like that. Here a group of muscles gets trained to a greater degree than those in the other parts of the body.

For the elderly, core stabilization is of prime importance. The aim of strength training includes improving the muscle-fiber size and contractile strength and increasing tendon and ligament strength. While prevention of injury, which is the muscle and connective tissue damage, is the primary aim, many bodybuilders do it to look good. And, they will by the time they finish their strength training program. Strengthening of the core helps the individual move around with ease and decreases the stress on the skeletal system. This prevents the person from getting tired during the day. During weight training, all muscles get strengthened. A typical workout consists of one set of treadmills for 10-15 minutes, 4 sets of dumbbell rows of 5 minutes, front squats using a rack machine 3 sets of 8 - 10 reps each, chest press, and pushups. You might like to add pull-ups and more dumbbell exercises, and you can do that as you go along. The conventional method tells you to push the limits, sweat it out until you cannot go on anymore. Well, that is okay, that is the way to develop muscles. But it is a huge strain! Check the BFR method and see how it compares to this.

The Simplicity of the BFR Method of Strength Training

People also refer to BFR training as occlusion training. The term occlusion refers to blocking or excluding a part of the blood flow to a working limb or body part. We see three parts of BFR - one is the occlusion, the second is the decreased weights, and the third is the increased reps.

Importance of occlusion.

Occlusion is the basis for BFR, it helps the user achieve a great deal more for a lot less. It shows remarkable results for muscle hypertrophy and strength. People with Parkinson's disease show great recovery within weeks of rehab with BFR. Studies carried out on the safety aspect showed a remarkable degree of safety present in the BFR process. The most important consideration was that of coagulation resulting in blood clot formation. Research showed we have a reduced risk of blood clotting when using BFR. The joint stress and tissue damage remain decreased because one uses light weights. Occlusion through the use of elastic bands helps you preserve body tissue when you exercise.

Ease of use.

Unlike conventional training methods, BFR uses easy-to-use methods. The first is the preference for smaller weights which helps even invalids and older people use them for their recovery process. We can fight most of the diseases and ailments better when the body is in good shape meaning the muscles are in top condition and responsive to the slightest impulse.
This is because the energy needed to move the arms and legs is less, so the person has enough surplus energy to respond to metabolic and other internal activities. More importantly, BFR doesn't stress the person out and one needn't use their entire body power at all.

Effectiveness through increased reps.

This method uses increased reps right from the word go. Since the weights are light, they are easy to do but the increased reps make up for this. In the place where one will make 10 reps one does 30 reps. The muscle becomes exhausted after the usual 10 reps and everything you do after that is a bonus. The body thinks it is 'overdoing' the exercise and responds accordingly.
It sends increased blood flow and growth nutrients to compensate. This allows the muscle cells in the region to develop much more than it normally would. You must use occlusion for each of the body parts by tying the extremities with an elastic band.

Chapter 3: Benefits

Exercising is the way of supplementing body energy by enhancing muscle power. Energy remains stored in the muscle fibers and supplies it to the body when needed. BFR increases this myriad times because the volume of the muscle mass is enormous. Muscles will not grow because we eat an enhanced diet alone, it needs the proper physical input in the form of an exercise regimen.

When your body exhausts other sources of energy it will begin to use the energy from the muscles. When this happens, the person will begin to lose muscle mass. The body uses carbohydrates from food in normal circumstances, but it can convert fat and proteins into energy when the need arises. This is why you need big muscles; it stores energy that helps you remain energized under all conditions. When you use BFR techniques, muscles grow extra big.

Specific Advantages of BFR Method

BFR has the name KAATSU training in Japan, the place where it originated. Dr. Sato is living proof of the efficacy of his method, his phenomenal muscle growth stands him in good stead even at his advanced age of 73. Other advantages of this innovative method are these:

- You can exercise with little or no weights even and this helps decrease injury risks.

- The low-load BFR control group showed better progress in functional capacity leading to better rehabilitation.

Sarcopenia is an age-related disease that leads to the loss of muscle and muscle strength. This is due to the deterioration of the quality of mitochondria lying within each cell of our body. In the past years, conventional methods of resistance training helped in preventing sarcopenia. The use of BFR helps older people keep their muscles intact with minimal effort.

Physiology Involved in BFR

The increase in muscle girth is easy because of two things. One is the establishment of blood vessels around the site of the original muscle fibers and the other is the stimulation of growth factors that helps secretion of hormones. The improvement of strength remains accompanied by an increase in the protein content due to the growth factors. This allows the muscles to store more energy.

1. Increase in muscle hypertrophy
2. The action of mechanical tension
   a. Cell swelling
   b. Release of hormones
   c. Activation of myogenic stem cells
   d. Hypoxia

Action of Restriction

In BFR, we create a hypoxic environment by occluding the flow of venous blood using a cuff. The cuff must remain proximal to the muscle which we exercise at the time. When blood flow increases in the region of the targeted tissues muscle hypertrophy occur. An increase in lactic acid and protons triggers low-oxygen conditions.

The anabolic response to this is the stimulation of twitch muscle response. This set of muscles responds fast to low-intensity exercises unlike the slow response Type I muscles that we target during conventional exercises. The elastic band pushes blood into the muscle tissues and traps it there. This is not possible in conventional methods.

Even otherwise, the targeted muscles in the conventional method are Type I that will not work when the oxygen gets depleted. The elastic band will only restrict the blood flow to a small extent so there is enough flow to bring in the blood to the area.

Increased Growth of Muscle Cells

Muscle hypertrophy occurs due to the interruption of regular cell growth and altered conditions in the tissues. An increase in the rate of cell growth begins when you stimulate it through rapid low-intensity reps. In the myofibers, between the plasma membrane and basal lamina, we find myogenic stem cells. Usually, they remain inactive but become responsive when we suffer an injury or there is an increase in mechanical tension. Under increased tension conditions, the stimulation of the stem cells helps increase muscle cell growth.

Cell swelling action.

When the water reaches the activated muscle cells, it causes them to swell. Water is necessary to cure conditions of increased tension and hormone levels. This improves the growth of the cells in a short time. The action takes place on the Type II cells that bear the tension in hypoxic conditions.

Increase in anaerobic metabolic activity.

During the training of the muscles, we see compression of blood vessels. The drop in the oxygen level activates hypoxia-inducible factor. This leads to an increase in the anaerobic metabolic activity which, in turn, causes lactic acid levels to rise. Due to the anaerobic activity, the glucose molecule splits into two lactic acid molecules. While we do not notice the presence of lactic acid under normal conditions if their levels rise above a specific amount the pain builds up. We can feel the 'burn' when we exercise.

The main result of this type of increase in anaerobic activity is that the Type I muscle fibers that need oxygen to work, stop working. Type II muscles now take up the brunt of the exercise leading to growth and expansion of muscle cells. KAATSU training with very light weights produces a profusion of muscle cells in about half the time it takes to produce the same effect using conventional methods.

Changes in activity at the cellular level.

Release of hormones occurs when we indulge in physical activity or the body detects an extended change in tension in the muscles. We witness an increase in collagen synthesis due to these growth hormones and insulin-like growth factors. This is mainly to help in muscle recovery and doesn't play a direct part in muscle hypertrophy. The muscles get strengthened while the accumulation of hydrogen ions and lactate helps stimulate the release of more growth hormones. Another good thing that takes place is the way myostatin is down-regulated. Myostatin inhibits cell growth and so shutting it down helps to improve the muscle hypertrophy process. The cell swelling activates the myogenic stem cells due to the mechanical tension.

Wow! Congratulations!

Do you know that **67%** of the readers **don't finish** the book they are reading and that a relevant percentage **don't even start the second chapter**?
You are on the good track to finish this useful practical guide and my family and I congratulate you for this! :)

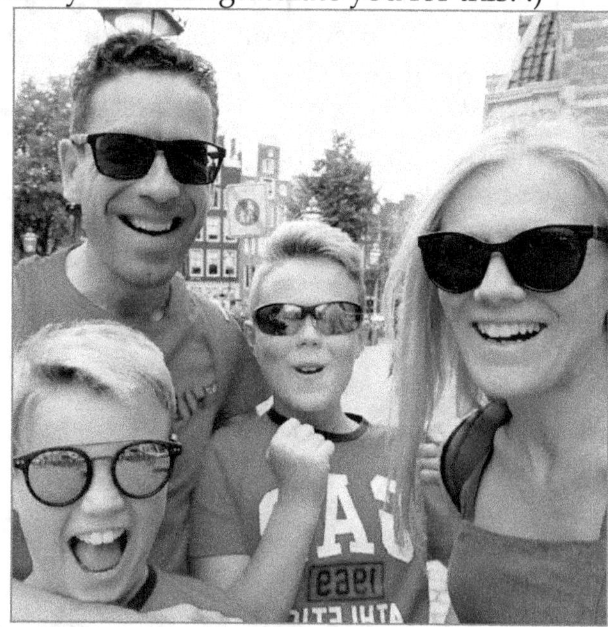

In fact, this book is fully practical with no fluff and I spent many cups of coffee to put it together.
Hope you like it and please leave a review in order to help me as an author and to improve the content of this book.
Your review is very important. I will read it very carefully as it will be used as a tool to refine my work! Thank you!

CLICK HERE TO LEAVE FEEDBACK ON AMAZON
If you're undecided, just leave the review later...

Ah! By the way, this photo was taken last Summer in Amsterdam. Very hot day! :)

Chapter 4: Workout Training Protocol and Correct Posture

The most important thing in BFR is to individualize the procedure for each person. As workout procedure depends on the individual, care about the restrictive blood flow remains important. Each person has a different physique, body type and weight, age, and physical condition. You need to apply immobilizations and training adaptations as needed.

Determine the Cuff Pressure

While applying the cuff to the limb one has to choose the right pressure. Higher pressures remain linked to higher risks and so it is usual to choose a lower, safer pressure. Limb Occlusion Pressure is the least pressure needed for a limb at a specific time and applied at a specific part of the limb. This stops the arterial blood flow distal to the cuff, lower pressures mean lower risk and pain. Occlusion Pressure (OP) is specific to each person, it is best to use the lowest cuff pressure that stops the blood flow to the needed amount.

A wide pneumatic cuff (say 10 cm) distributes a lower pressure of 50 mmHg/cm when you apply a pressure of 250 mmHg. The use of thinner cuffs will result in higher pressures and since we don't wish to cut the blood flow completely, it is not advisable to opt for higher pressures. The cuff gets tied to the limb along with a pressure valve.

Dimensions of the cuff.

The length of the cuff for the arm is 17¼" and the width is 2" and for the leg, the cuff is 29¼" long and 3" wide. In the absence of a regulation cuff, you could use an elastic band.

List of Exercises to Do

Dumbbell Flat Chest Press

Put on the bands near the shoulder joint of your arm and lie down on the bench. and do the first set of reps. Say this is 35 after you finish this set you wait for 30 seconds. Then, you do 20 reps and take rest for 30 seconds. Do one more set of 20 reps and rest for 30 seconds. Finish with one last set of 15 reps and then rest for 30 seconds. Loosen the bands and rest for one minute. This completes your first cycle. Do two cycles. (35 - 30, 20 - 30, 20 - 30, 15 -30; 1 minute - repeat once).

Weights to use.

Do not use the usual max weight of 180 lbs. but opt for 30-50% of this. The conventional weight trainers use 120 lbs. which is 60-70% of the max. In BFR, you need to use only 60lbs. Do the reps fully as this is important.

Adjust the cuff pressure.

The pneumatic air cuffs allow arterial blood flow. The blood returning to the heart, the venous flow gets stopped completely. Make sure you do not stop the arterial flow completely because you want the blood to flow into the arm and saturate it while you exercise.

The method of chest press.

Once you are horizontal on the bench, lower the bar with the right weights on to your chest. Your fists must come down and go up straight all the time. One rep is when you have completed one up and down movement of the bar. Keep the bar near the rest so that you can keep it back once you have completed the reps.

Dumbbell Incline Chest Press

The method of exercise is the Incline Chest Press is the same
as the previous only you keep the bench inclined and then lie
down on it. The number of reps is 15 -30, 15 -30, 15 -30. Then,
rest for one minute and do one more cycle. Use the cuffs like
before and make sure there is enough blood flow into the arm.

Do Push-ups

This simple but effective exercise for body fitness becomes
more effective when you use cuffs. Put the cuffs on your arm
and adjust the pressure valves until the blood is flowing into
the arm but it is not flowing out. You will get the hang of this
with practice.
Lay down on the floor with your face down and keep your
hands below your chest. Keep your legs stiff and straight
when you do the pushups. Do 30 reps and wait for 30 seconds,
then do 20 more and wait for 30 seconds. Do the second one,
two more times (30 -30, 20 -30, 20 -30, 20 -30).

Chest Flyes

Remember to put your air cuffs (or elastic bands) before you
begin the exercise. In BFR, this is the most important thing
because otherwise, it will be only plain conventional
exercising.
In Chest Flyes, we use dumbbells and lie down on the bench.
To begin the rep, we start with the dumbbells straight up and
bring the hands down on either side until they are horizontal.
Then, we move them up until they are horizontal again. That
is one rep.

Use light 5 lbs. dumbbell and not standard 8 or 10 lbs.
dumbbells. Do 20 reps to start and take 20 seconds rest. Then,
do three rounds of 15 reps and 20 seconds rest (20 - 20, 15 - 20,
15 - 20, 15 - 20; 1-minute rest. Repeat the cycle).

This exercise is good for developing the chest and arm
muscles. Do one set while warming up and another while
warming down.

One Arm Row

This is an exercise for the arm. Tie the cuff to the arm like
before. We use the bench like before. Put one arm and one leg
on the bench. Rest your other leg beside it and take the
dumbbell in your hand.
Move the arm up and down in the given number of reps. Do
30 reps and rest for 30 seconds. Then, do three sets of 20 reps
with 30 seconds rest each (30 - 30, 20 - 30, 20 - 30, 20 - 30; 1
minute - repeat once).
Then, repeat for the other hand in the same way. This exercise
helps build strength in the upper arms and wrists. Make sure
you don't move your elbows away from your body while
exercising.

Leg Curl

In this exercise, two sets of muscles remain targeted, the calf
muscles and the hamstrings. You will need specialized
equipment for this. It is an inclined bench that has a provision
for you to lie down on it and rest your thighs comfortably.
You bend your legs back and you can adjust the weight that
you lift with the legs.

Bend your legs back so that the weights get lifted and then release them by straightening your legs. This will be one rep. Do 25 reps and rest for 20 seconds. Then, do three sets of 20 reps with 20 seconds rest each, this will complete one cycle. Release the elastic bands and rest for one full minute. Then, repeat the entire cycle (25 -20, 20 -20, 20 -20, 20 -20; 1 minute - repeat once).

Tie the bands close to the top of the leg and keep the pressure at 30% of LOP. Take off the bands after each cycle. This exercise is useful for long-distance runners and sprinters.

Dumbbell Curls

The best thing about dumbbell curls is that besides adding strength to the upper arms, it makes the wrist supple. You target the biceps and if you opt for the barbell bicep curl you get more strength in your arms. But, that doesn't mean you shouldn't do the alternating dumbbell curl which is less strenuous.

When you do the BFR curl, choose light dumbbells (usual weight is 80 pounds for men and 40 pounds for women in conventional weight training) about 20 -30 lbs. would do fine. The lesser weight helps you do more reps with ease. Tie your elastic band around your forearm so that you find your palm area remains red and doesn't remain white for more than half a second (check the test for BFR band pressure test given in this book).

There are two parts in the bicep muscles - short and long head. The way you hold your dumbbell allows you to target the short or the long head. A supinated grip (wrist faces forward or upward) lets you target the short head while a pronated grip targets the long head. Make sure you use both grips alternately.

One upward movement followed by one downward
movement of the dumbbell is one rep. Use a supinated grip
for one cycle and the next, use a pronated grip. Do 20 reps
with 20 second s rest three times (20 -20, 20 - 20, 20 -20; 1-
minute rest - change grip, repeat cycle).
Keep an eye on the elastic band so that it doesn't become very
tight. Allow enough blood flow into the muscle (arterial
blood), it is the venous blood that you need to stop. You can
check the tightness by testing the redness of your palm).

Overhead Dumbbell Extension

This exercise targets the triceps region of the arms. The thing
to note is that when you raise the dumbbell is your elbows
open up, the weight is too much. If this is so, use a lower
weight. Other than that, make sure you use a straight back,
this is to prevent any unwanted sprain to the back.
Take the dumbbell (usual weight for conventional resistance
training is 20 lbs.) that is 8 lbs. or even 4 lbs. for BFR training.
Tie the bands (remember to loosen them after you finish one
cycle) and check that the blood flow is present. Do 15 - 20
cycles, that is, 15 reps with 20 seconds rest, thrice (15 -20, 15 -
20, 15 -20, 1-minute rest - repeat cycle). Untie the band and
rest for one full minute. This helps reduce the risks and so
don't neglect this part. Then, do the repeat cycle.
Sit in a straight-back chair (or bench) and bring the dumbbell
up above your head. Grasp it with both hands and lower the
dumbbell behind your back. Your elbows must remain close
to your body otherwise change the weights, make them less.
Bring the weight back up. This will make one rep. Be sure to
remove the band after you finish one cycle during your rest
period.

Quarter Squat

In a quarter squat, you don't have to bend your knees to 90°
since this is a quarter squat. It is enough to bend your knees to
45° and so it is possible to lift more weights in a quarter squat.
When you do the quarter squat in BFR training, you need to
lift even lesser weights. So, instead of doing 200 lbs. you only
got to do 60 lbs.
Make sure to fix the BFR bands if you have them or else use
elastic bands. Check the pressure by pressing on your palm
and see if the color comes back within one second. If not, the
band is too tight. Loosen it a little.
Load the bar with two 30 lbs. weights, lift it and rest it on your
shoulders. Spread your legs until it is as wide as your
shoulders. Keep your back straight. Bend your knees in a
squat and bring the weight down. When your knees remain
bent at 45° rise so that you are standing erect once again. This
represents one rep.
Do 30 reps and rest for 20 seconds. Be sure that the knees do
not go beyond your toes when you squat. The next rep will be
20 followed by 20 seconds rest. Do this once more so that the
cycle becomes as 30 -20, 20 -20, 20 -20, 1-minute rest - repeat
once).

Stiff-Legged Deadlift

When you do the leg curls, your lower and mid hamstrings
get strengthened. Here you work with the upper part of your
leg. One must try not to involve the back too much. Also, this
helps you work out your hips.

- Bend your knees a little and move your feet until it is
  shoulder-width apart.

- Stand with the weight on your heels, inhale and bend without stretching your back.
- Let your arms holding the dumbbell down until it is below the knee level.
- Keep your back straight, don't hunch your back. Look forward as you do the exercise.
- One rep will consist of one downward move and the follow up upward movement.

Do 25 reps and keep the weight light say 8 pounds. Tie your elastic or BFR band and keep the blood flowing all the time. After the reps, take a break for 20 seconds. Follow this up with two more cycles of 20 -20 type that is 20 reps and 20 seconds rest. Then, loosen your bands and rest for one minute. Repeat the cycle once more. The entire entire process is 25 - 20, 20 -20, 20 - 20, 1 minute - repeat once.

Chapter 5: Risks and contradictions

Our existence with BFR is a glorious affair, one that remains tempered with care and diligence. Since it caters to a wide range of users such as the healthy and those recovering from injury, the young and the old, those wishing to prevent sarcopenia, the age-related loss of muscle, and those who wished to add strength to their body frames. The use of BFR brought all these fitness enthusiasts together but there were risks as with all other forms of physical activity.

Plus points of BFR.

Keeping the weights light lessens the risks considerably but even then, many conditions will prevent one from working using BFR. It takes at least three sessions of BFR before your body begins to adjust to it. The smaller weights help the elderly and the injured patients undergoing physiotherapy because they do not have to lift a huge weight to get benefits.

Set the Safe BFR Band Pressure

The process begins by establishing the LOP (Limb Occlusion Pressure) of the patient while he or she is lying, sitting, and standing. Now, they go through the medical history to make sure there are no contraindications.

Check for contraindications.

The process is safe if you do it properly but when you use a cuff system that is rigid you face risks such as a stroke or heart attack from hypertension and lethal blood clots. The factors that could add to the risks are these:

- Long travel - After a long journey, you should avoid doing the BFR exercise. After a few days, your body condition will stabilize. Pooling and blood stasis increase risks.
- Being bedridden - Being bedridden will also increase the risks in the same way.
- Blood stasis - When the blood has undergone occlusion recently as is the case after surgery, the risk will be more. This is due to clotting.
- Cardiovascular risk - People with heart problems need to clear the exercise program with their doctor. Start exercising only after he has cleared high-intensity exercise.
- Damage to blood vessel - When there is a limb injury, it could increase the risk factor. This might occur after a venous graft for instance. The risk also increases when

the circulation is poor. If this is the case, one has to start with lighter weights.

If a person has high blood pressure, it is better to opt for exercises without weights. You can do squats and single-joint exercises.

More Contraindications and Rare Side Effects

1. Condition of rhabdomyolysis - Rhabdomyolysis can cause kidney failure and cardiac arrhythmia. It happens due to the presence of intracellular contents that occur when there is damage to the muscle. It might happen when one exercises with very heavy weights. When doing KAATSU exercises, it is important to remember to use light weights.

2. Condition of hemodialysis - When one undergoes hemodialysis, they will have arteriovenous fistulas. Doing blood flow restriction will increase the risks considerably.

3. Condition of mastectomy - Women who had mastectomy must avoid BFR until they recover completely.

4. Use of beta-alanine supplements - One must avoid beta-alanine supplements when you indulge in BFR training. Beta-alanine increases homeostasis in tissues and doing BFR will interrupt this process.

Use of BFR for the Elderly

Age-related muscle loss is a reality that you address with BFR. This condition can begin at a young age. One must take proactive steps to prevent this and if you go ahead without intervention, you can lose up to 6 lbs. in one decade.

Muscle maintenance problems.

Fast-twitch fibers get activated by blood flow restriction training. You can get around this with a high-intensity interval (HIIT) training regime. The human growth hormone gets released by this exercise regime. Elderly people enjoy this because of the lower weights used.

In the elderly, the use of BFR will help restore functionality and it doesn't need any extensive effort to regain mobility and freedom. It is low risk leading Dr. Sato to call it anti-aging medicine." Studies have proved BFR is effective in activating stem cells. It helps change fast-twitch fibers into oxidative fibers, improves bone repair and growth.

Need for separate exercises for ligaments and tendons.

It is not proven yet whether ligaments and tendons get strengthened when one does blood flow restriction training. The absence of heavy loads may mean that the muscles will become strong but the tendons may not. You will need to do a separate set of exercises to strengthen the connective tissues.

Reflection on KAATSU

Being one of the most useful exercise strategies, most people including the old and the injured would prefer to add KAATSU training to their regular exercise routine if they could. Besides helping preserve muscle and bone mass, it has the added advantage of using light weights making your exercises easy to perform. This also decreases the risks.
The logic and science behind restricted blood flow training are simple and impressive. It is enough to do this exercise thrice a week and alternate between the hands and legs so that the benefits remain divided between both. The elastic knee wraps give you the advantage of covering a larger area with their bigger width and along with their elasticity, they provide good protection against risk. Also, the probability of the band sliding down is less.
If you use rubber tubing or straps made of nylon can restrict the blood flow. It will also reduce your flexibility.

The Action of BFR on the Cardiovascular System

Assuming that one has got clearance to exercise from one's physician, or supposing that you are a healthy individual, it is natural that one wishes to include BFR into the regular exercise routine. Read about their action on the nervous and cardiovascular system below.

One branch of thinking believes that restricted blood flow can damage veins and so it will be bad in the long run. Studies show something else. Over a month's time, we see that the ability of the vessel to vasodilate increases. There is an increase in the blood flow when compared to that of conventional resistance training. Also, in the conventional resistance training where you use 70-80% LOP, there is a doubling of arterial blood pressure and heart rates reach the biggest value.

Compared to this, the low-intensity BFR shows an increase in the heart rate and blood pressure only up to 11-12% which is much lower than the one we saw before. We understand the significant difference that is we apply only 50-220 mmHg when we use BFR. During conventional high-intensity exercises, the contraction of the muscles can create pressures in the muscles that are about 500 mmHg, and, at times, we see it touch 1000 mmHg.

One must realize that occlusion occurs in traditional resistance training even for moderate forces. We see a smaller version of this in BFR.

Dealing with Blood Clots

The other big worry about BFR is that thrombosis might occur because of it. The term refers to the formation of blood clots that block the blood flow inside blood vessels. We understand the effect of BFR when we study the factors that influence the formation of blood clots.

a) Vascular damage

b) Hyper ability to form blood clots

c) Vascular occlusion of the flow of blood

One has to know that clot formation is an intermediate state caused by imbalance existing between breaking down process and coagulation. Studies show that low-intensity BFR doesn't increase coagulation. But, it may break down clots on an increasing scale. For all normal uses, BFR is perfectly safe. The only thing one has to remember is to not occlude the blood flow completely but keep it at 40-50% to increase the benefits.

BFR and the Nervous System

One common concern among BFR users is whether BFR affects the nervous system and in what way. There was a small percentage of users who experienced numbness in the limbs. But, further studies over an extended four-week period saw no change in their nerve impulse speeds.

Chapter 6: BFR Equipment

Rather than ordering by approximation, one should order by measurement. The smart cuff size will be accurate when you use the actual body measurement. Smart cuff size gets graded 1 to 5 and depends on the circumference measured between your shoulder and the bicep. This is for the upper body measurement.

Picking the Right Size Cuff

For the lower body measurement, the measurement of your thigh nearest to the hip If the size is between two sizes, go with the lower value.

The Limb Size in Inches	Smart Cuff Size
6 - 11	1
11 - 16	2
16 - 22	3
22 - 29	4
29 - 38	5

You will need two cuffs, one for the upper body and another for the lower. Place the cuff on the proximal part between the bicep and deltoid for the arm and the proximal part of the thigh or femur for the leg.

Working with the cuff.

The bladder system with a single chamber allows the user to make use of the Limb Occlusion Pressure (LOP) as an indicator of the needed pressure we need to set in the cuff. Standard cuffs are 4" wide will keep the operating pressure within safe limits. You get the inflation metrics on each cuff according to its size. The cuff inflation has enough freedom of movement along with a stable tube detachment in the valve system that gives you consistent results.

In every set, you get four cuffs and one mesh bag. You can use the hand gauge to measure the pressure before beginning your exercise cycle. After you have applied your cuff you can check the pressure by using a simple field method. Press below the thumb area in your palm until it becomes white. Now, release the pressure and check how long it takes to become red again. If the time is less than one second, then your band is set right. If the time is more than three seconds, then the band is probably set too tight. Also, make sure you do not experience any numbness or tingling. If you get a pinkness or redness in your palm, then you are ready to start exercising.

You can get the latest KAATSU original equipment which doesn't cost much. It costs $900 - $1,200 but you can also get inexpensive brands for as little as $25 - $40. The drawback with the cheaper versions is that you can't do KAATSU cycling and must learn to set the pressure by yourself.

Chapter 7: Where to Buy Equipment

Just search for "blood flow restriction" in Amazon and pick the best reviewed products.

Below I give you a few recommendations with my affiliate Amazon links. They won't cost you anything more, but the commission does help to fill my coffee fund and keep me writing – so thanks if you do ;)

Blood Flow Restriction Cuffs (BFR) Training Therapy Occlusion Restriction Cuffs with mmHg Monitor and Pump

Occlusion Training Bands

Vikingstrength Occlusion Blood Resistance Bands for Arms and Legs

Stargoods Occlusion Bands, Restriction of Blood Flow Muscle Straps Training

Occlusion Training Bands, Rigid Edition

Conclusion

For all people involved in sports training, rehabilitation therapy, and improvement of general fitness, BFR training provides the best window of opportunity to get strength in your muscles and do so without exerting yourself with extensive weights. Now that you are at the end of this book, *"BFR: Blood Flow Restriction,"* you must have gained valuable insight into the working of BFR training and the modalities needed to get the best benefit.

You are ready to take on the world, show your muscles to the people who care. Develop them using BFR and be there in the limelight.

Here is Wishing You the Very Best on Your Road to Absolute Fitness with BFR!

Thank you!

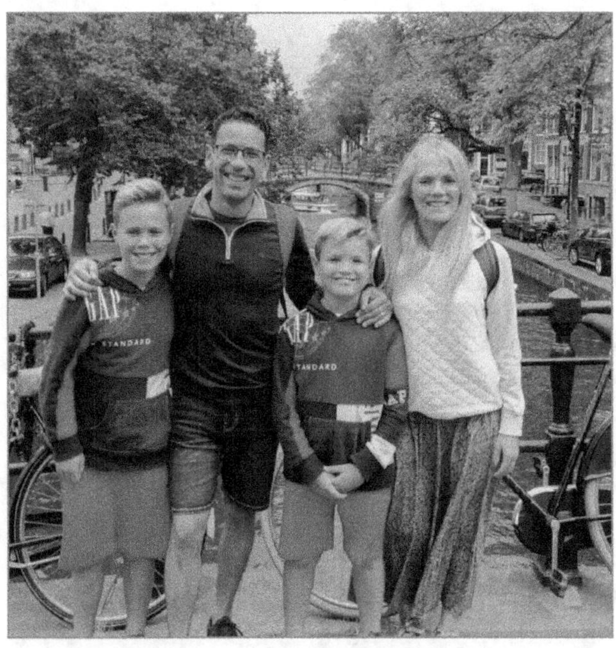

Hope you liked the book and please reread/study it!
Please leave a review in order to help me as an author and to improve and refine the content of this book.
Your review is very important. I will read it very carefully as it will be used as a tool to deliver better books! Many thanks in advance!
Please go to your account on Amazon or click on the link below.

[CLICK HERE TO LEAVE A REVIEW ON AMAZON!](#)

Thank you and good luck! Cheers!

Bibliography

- Douris, P. C., Cogen, Z. S., Fields, H. T., Greco, L. C., Hasley, M. R., Machado, C. M., ... DiFrancisco-Donoghue, J. (2018, April). THE EFFECTS OF BLOOD FLOW RESTRICTION TRAINING ON FUNCTIONAL IMPROVEMENTS IN AN ACTIVE SINGLE SUBJECT WITH PARKINSON DISEASE. Retrieved from https://www.ncbi.nlm.nih.gov/pmc/articles/PMC606305 5/

- Mandel, E. R. (2011). *Changes in conduit artery blood flow and diameter post blood flow restriction*. Waterloo, Ont.: University of Waterloo.

- Blood Flow Restricted Resistance Training In Older Adults. (2015). *The Gerontologist, 55*(Suppl_2), 144–144. doi: 10.1093/geront/gnv517.04

www.ingramcontent.com/pod-product-compliance
Lightning Source LLC
Chambersburg PA
CBHW050749250726

48662CB00005B/2113